# "WHAT'S HAPPENING TO ME?"

Books in this delightful series . . .

"WHERE DID I COME FROM?" by Peter Mayle and Arthur Robins. The facts of life without any nonsense and with illustrations.

"WHERE DID I COME FROM?" African-American Edition. The classic about sex and birth, illustrated for African Americans.

"WHAT'S HAPPENING TO ME?" by Peter Mayle and Arthur Robins. A guide to puberty, from the authors of "WHERE DID I COME FROM?"

"WHY AM I GOING TO THE HOSPITAL?" by Claire Ciliotta, Carole Livingston and Dick Wilson. A helpful guide to a new experience.

"WHY WAS I ADOPTED?" by Carole Livingston and Arthur Robins. The facts of adoption with love and illustrations.

"WHAT AM I DOING IN A STEPFAMILY?" by Claire Berman and Dick Wilson. How two families can be better than one.

HOW TO BE A PREGNANT FATHER by Peter Mayle and Arthur Robins. An illustrated survival guide for the father-to-be.

Each book is delightfully written and illustrated in the style of the book you hold in your hands!

Ask for these books at your bookseller. If your bookseller can't supply you, order direct from the publisher by calling 1-800-221-2647. And send for our complete catalog of titles: Kensington Publishing Corp., 850 Third Avenue, New York, NY 10022.

You'll be glad you did!

# "WHAT'S HAPPENING TO ME?"

The answers to some of the world's most embarrassing questions.

Written by Peter Mayle.
Illustrated by Arthur Robins. Designed by Paul Walter.

Lyle Stuart
Kensington Publishing Corp.
www.kensingtonbooks.com

LYLE STUART books are published by

Kensington Publishing Corp.
850 Third Avenue
New York, NY 10022

All Kensington titles, imprints, and distributed lines are available at special quantity discounts for bulk purchases for sales promotions, premiums, fund raising, educational, or institutional use. Special book excerpts or customized printings can also be created to fit specific needs. For details, write or phone the office of the Kensington special sales manager: Kensington Publishing Corp., 850 Third Avenue, New York, NY 10022, attn: Special Sales Department, phone 1-800-221-2647.

First printing 1975

30  29  28  27  26  25

Printed in the United States of America

ISBN 0-8184-0312-8

Library of Congress Cataloging-in-Publication Data

Mayle, Peter.
   What's happening to me?
  SUMMARY; Discusses the mental and physical changes
  that take place during puberty.
  1. Puberty–Juvenile literature.  (1. Puberty.  2. Adolescence.)
  I. Robins, Arthur.  II. Title.
Qp84.4.M39            612.6′61              75–14410

This book is for all of you who are suffering from growing pains. We hope it brings some fast relief.

## Everybody goes through it.
## Nobody talks about it.

Don't let anyone fool you.

People say that your childhood and school days are about the happiest times of your life. That's not altogether true.

The years between ten and fourteen may be a lot of fun. But physically, they'll probably be among the most puzzling years of your life.

That's because you're turning from a child into a young adult. Big changes are taking place, both in your mind and your body.

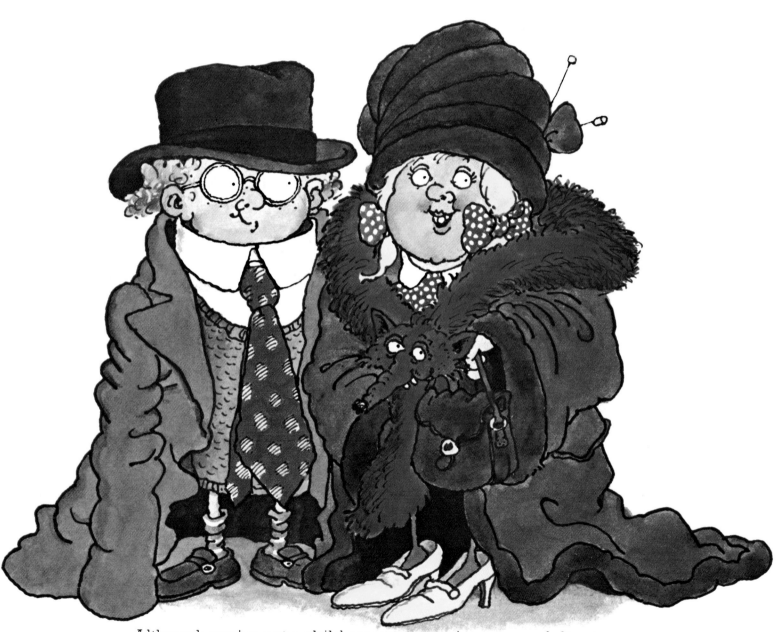

Although you're not a child any more, you're not an adult yet.
This book is about the time in between.

When they start to happen, it may be hard for you to understand and adjust to them. What makes it harder is that nobody talks about them very much.

Your parents may have forgotten what it was like to be your age and to have your problems. Teachers are often too busy teaching school to explain. And your friends (who may try to act sophisticated) usually don't know any more than you do.

This book can be very helpful to you.

It won't solve all your problems or even answer all your questions. But when you're through reading it, you should know a lot more about what's happening to you. And be a lot better prepared to cope with it.

We've tried to touch all the important bases. But if you still have unanswered questions, talk to people you can trust.

They can help. And you'll find if you're not embarrassed about asking the questions, they won't be embarrassed about giving you the answers.

A school teacher just doesn't have the time
to answer everybody's questions.

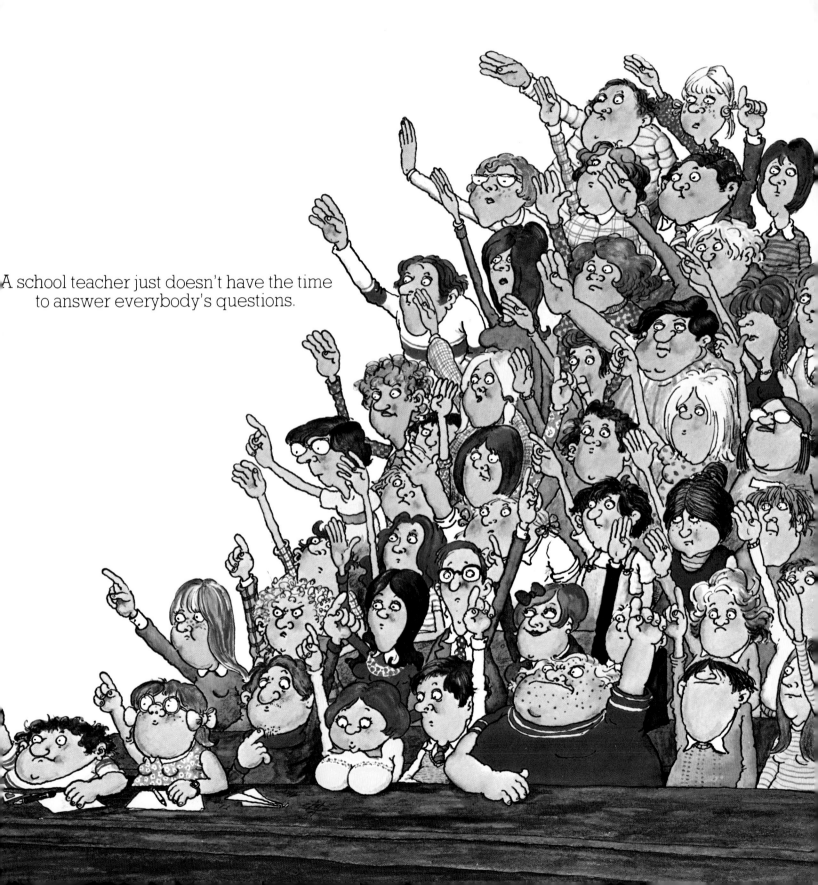

All the changes you're going through and will go through are quite normal. They're nothing to be ashamed of, and certainly nothing to be afraid of.

Remember that. Remember, too, that you're not the only one who has ever gone through this difficult time.

It happened to your parents. It happened to your heroes.

Most movie stars have had pimples. The best football player in the world probably worried when he was a boy because he didn't have much hair on his chest. And some of the most beautiful women were very homely as little girls.

Despite that, they all came through it pretty well. So will you.

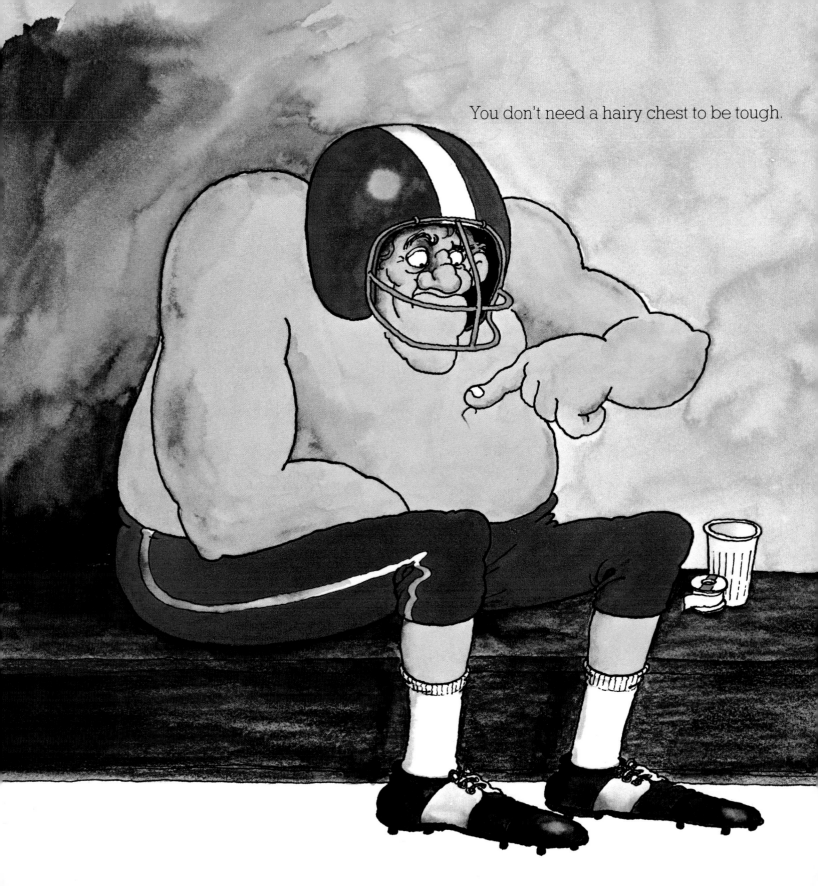

You don't need a hairy chest to be tough.

### Why you change.

The main reason you change is very simple. Nature changes you from a child into an adult so you can mate and reproduce the human species.

In other words, so that you can have children of your own.

The instinct to reproduce is common to all living things, from fleas to flowers to elephants.

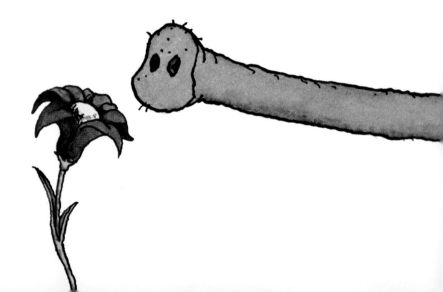

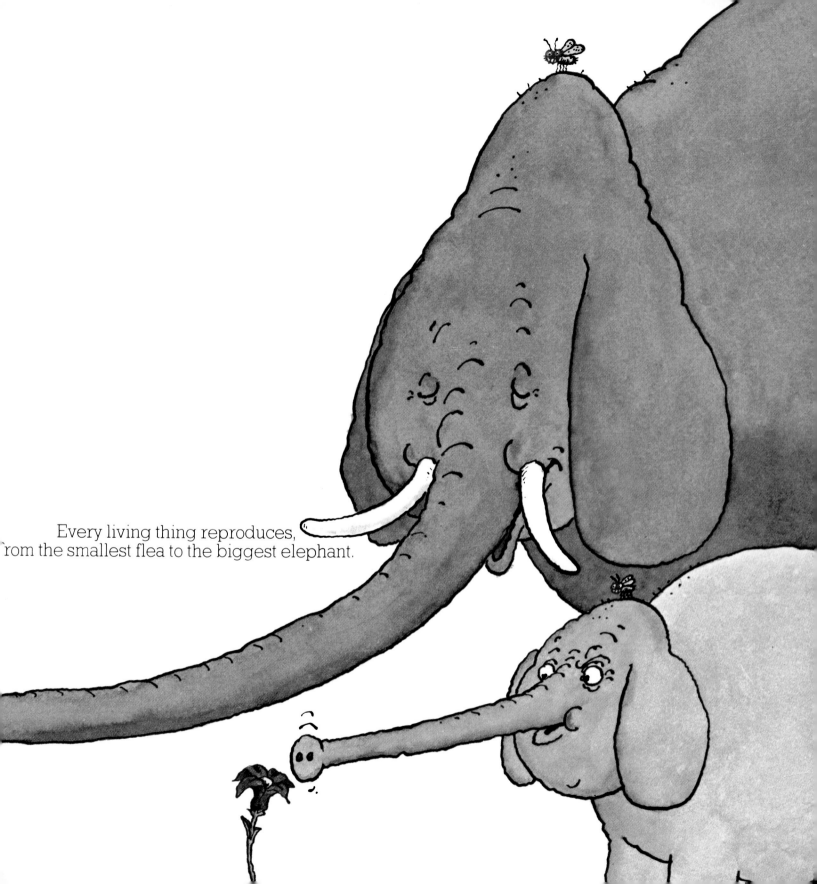

Every living thing reproduces,
from the smallest flea to the biggest elephant.

But it would be bad organiza-
tion on nature's part if you could
start having babies when you were
only five or six years old. (Imagine.
You could be a grandparent at the
age of twelve.)

So nature waits.

She begins the process some-
time during the years between ten
and thirteen. These years, called
the puberty years, are very busy
ones for both your mind and your
body. Many of the biggest changes
in your life begin to take place now.

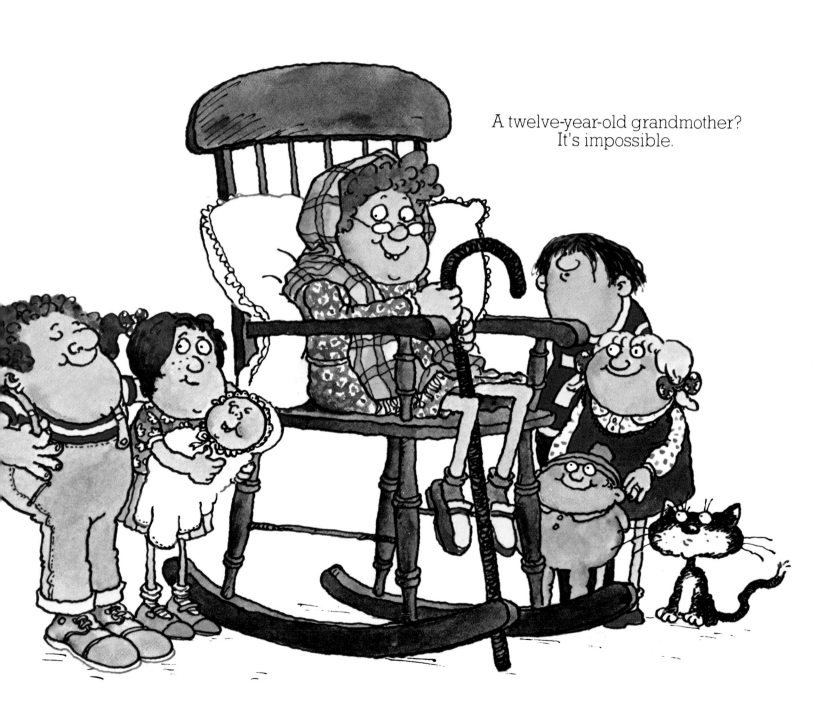

A twelve-year-old grandmother?
It's impossible.

## Is puberty catching?

No, it's not a disease. It's the medical name for the process we're describing: the change from child to adult.

Obviously, the changes a girl goes through are not the same changes that a boy goes through.

So to give you a clearer idea of what happens and when, we've done two charts.

Before you look at them, remember this; it's very important.

The changes that happen to the girl and the boy in this book won't happen to you at exactly the same age. We're all different, and we grow at different speeds.

With some of us, the changes start early. With some, they come later. You will change at different times than your friends. It doesn't mean you're any better or worse than they are. It just means you're you.

That's why you should only use these charts as a rough guide. Don't time yourself by them.

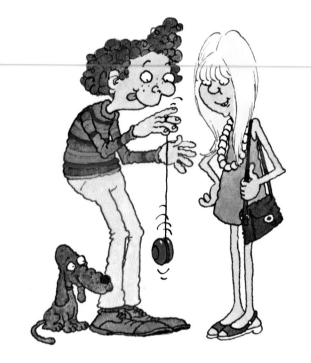

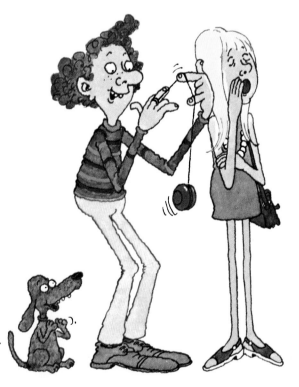

Often, but not always, girls grow up faster than boys.

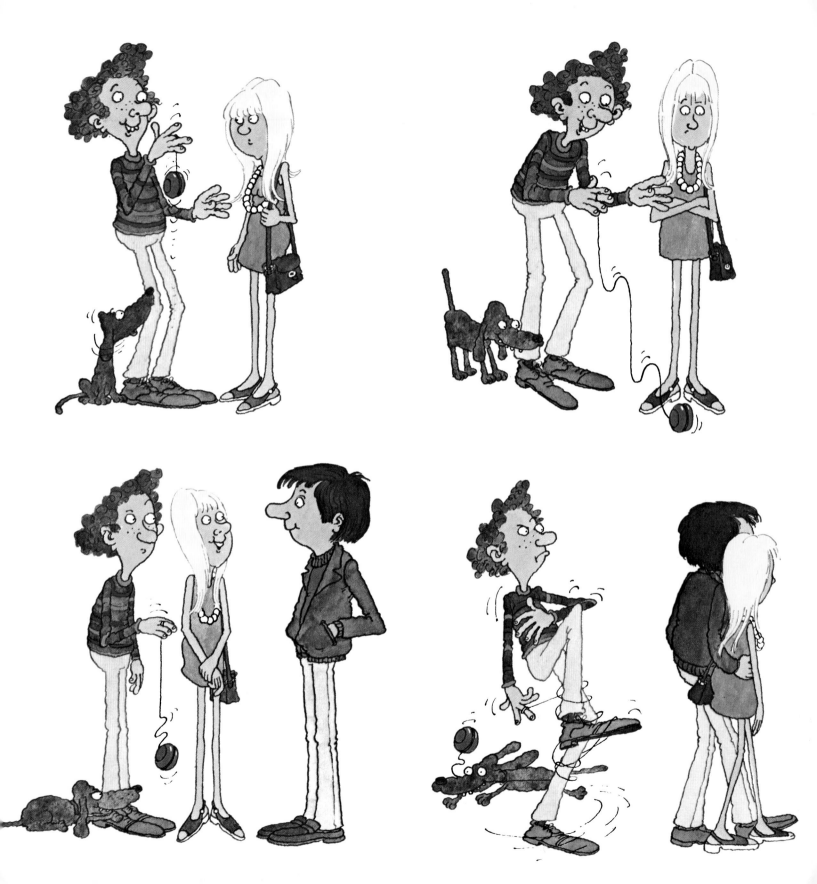

# Girl's Guide

### 8 to 10 years old.

Unless you're an early starter, puberty hasn't really begun yet. You don't have breasts or pubic hair, and most girls this age are not specially interested in boys.

### 11 to 12 years old.

Puberty gets going. Your breasts start to develop; nipples begin to stand out. Pubic hair makes its first appearance, and your hips become a little broader. Your voice may get slightly lower, and you may start to have periods.

### 13 to 14 years old.

This is often the age when you start having regular periods. You're not growing upwards quite as fast now, but your body is still busy. Pubic hair and breasts continue to flourish.

### 15 to 16 years old.

By now, your emotional life is probably in full swing, and boys have well and truly taken over as a major subject of interest. Along with that often comes an increase in your confidence.

### 17 to 18 years old.

You're now pretty much a young woman, and no longer a little girl. Breasts, pubic hair and hips have developed. Although your emotional development will continue, your physical development is just about complete.

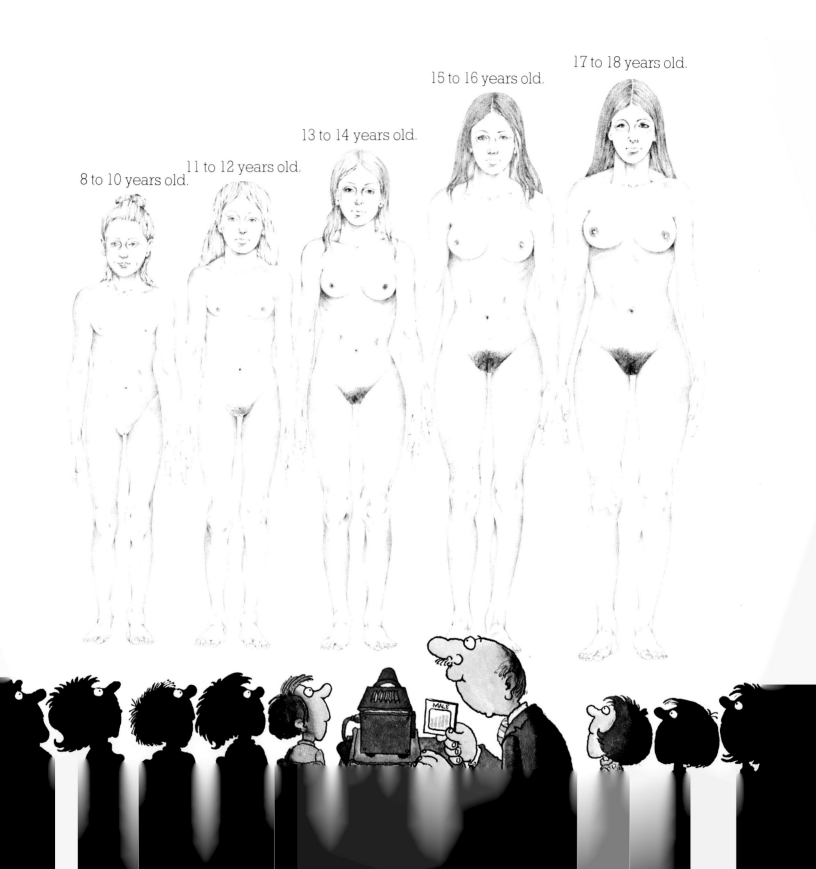

8 to 10 years old.

11 to 12 years old.

13 to 14 years old.

15 to 16 years old.

17 to 18 years old.

## Boy's Guide

8 to 10 years old.

As you can see, not a sign of pubic hair yet, and the penis is still quite small. Shoulders are slim, and the body shape is not too different from that of a little girl.

11 to 12 years old.

The hormone testosterone gets to work. You grow faster, your shoulders and chest become broader, your penis gets thicker and longer. Your voice may deepen too, but it generally doesn't break just yet.

13 to 14 years old.

Usually a very busy couple of years. Your first pubic hair, your first wet dream and the breaking of your voice could all happen around this age. Meanwhile, you're still growing fast.

15 to 16 years old.

Sadly, this is often the age of the pimple. The texture of your skin changes, and your sebaceous glands are producing so much oil you may get quite a few spots and blackheads.

17 to 18 years old.

By now, you're probably having to shave; if not every day, then once or twice a week. Your earlier interest in girls may now be concentrated on one special girl. Physically, you're a fully-developed man.

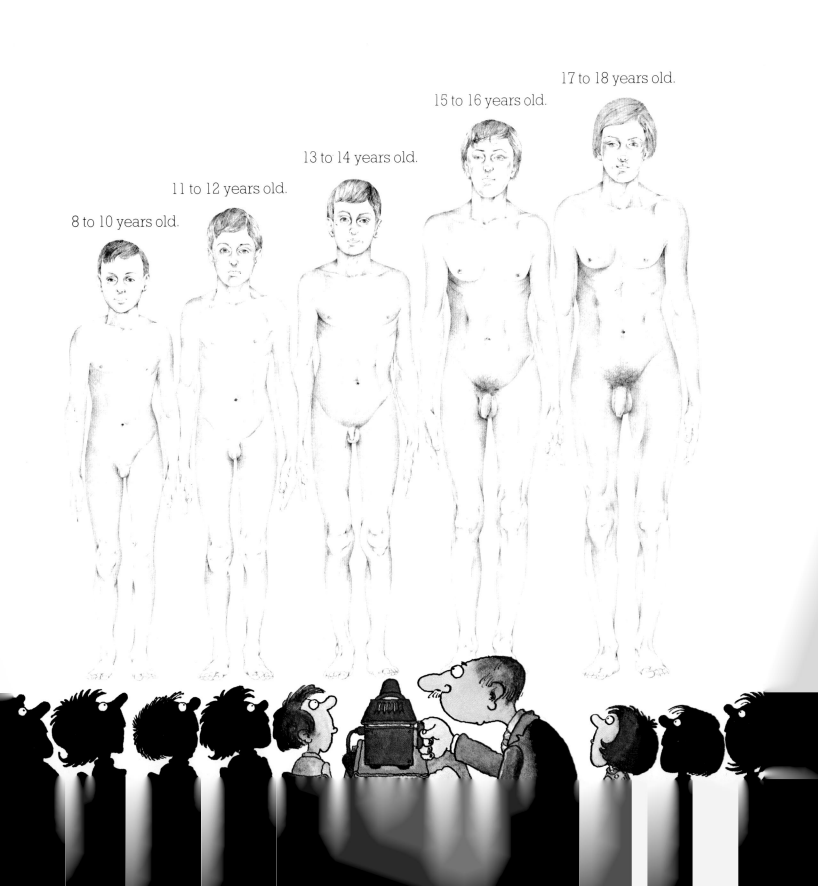

8 to 10 years old.

11 to 12 years old.

13 to 14 years old.

15 to 16 years old.

17 to 18 years old.

Right. Now that you've had a look at the charts, you're starting to find out what's happening to you.

We've explained some of the words and the changes in the pages that follow. And we've done it with questions and answers, because that seemed to be the most direct way to tell you what you want to know.

We call these the world's most embarrassing questions, because that's what they are. (At least, they were to us when we were your age.)

Try not to be embarrassed.
These changes happen to everyone.

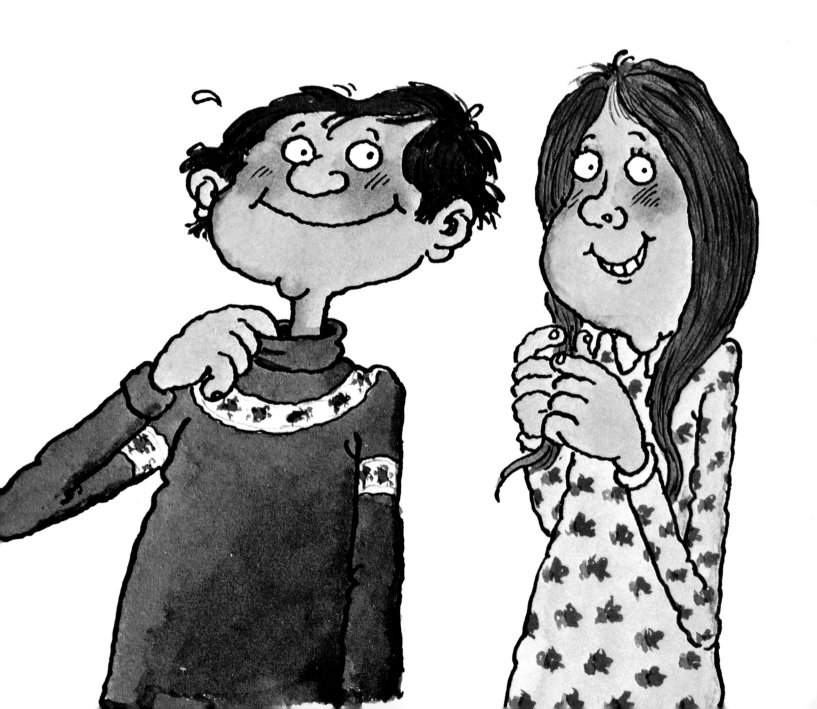

## But first, a word from your hormones.

Before going any further, it's high time you were introduced to your hormones. They're produced in organs in your body called glands. You never see them, so they're difficult to describe.

But they're very important. If you didn't have glands and hormones you wouldn't change into an adult.

The hormones we're talking about come in two sexes, just like people. And they have pretty fancy names. The female sex hormone is called estrogen. The male hormone is testosterone.

These two aren't the only hormones in your body by any means. But they're the ones to remember, because they're the ones that cause most of your physical changes.

And they're going to be very busy during the next few pages.

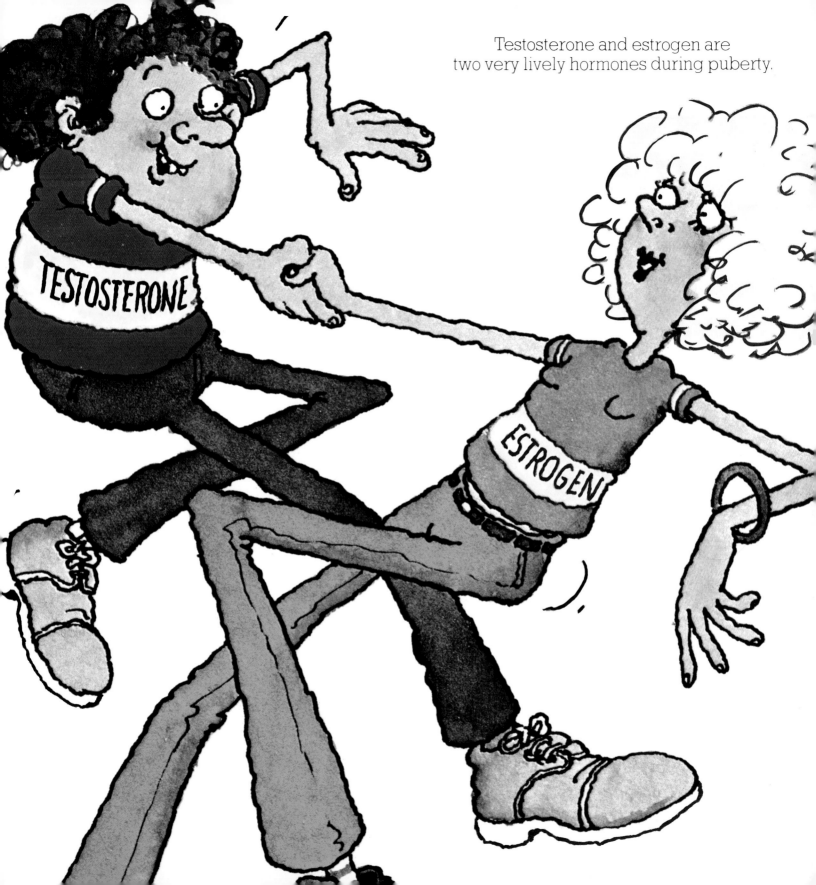

Testosterone and estrogen are two very lively hormones during puberty.

## The world's most embarrassing questions.

Some of these questions only apply to girls. Some only to boys.

We put them together because we thought you might like to know what happens to the opposite sex while you're going through your changes.

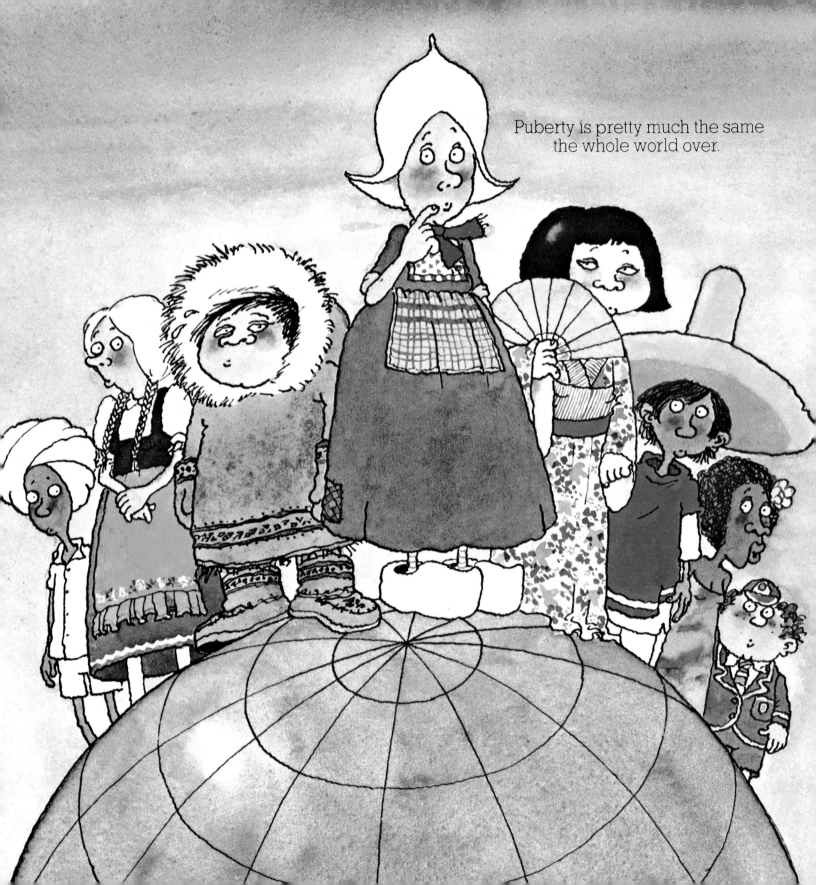

Puberty is pretty much the same the whole world over.

## "Why is my chest getting bumpy?"

If you're a girl, one day you'll look in the mirror and there they'll be. Two distinct bumps, where before there was nothing but a flat expanse of chest.

(Incidentally, boys' breasts sometimes get slightly larger and a little tender during puberty. This is quite normal; it will disappear as the male hormones get to work.)

But for girls these bumps signal the beginnings of your breasts, and they might make you feel a little selfconscious until you've gotten used to having them.

Also, if your breasts develop early, some of your girl friends may try to make fun of you. Let it pass. Those "jokes" are usually caused by jealousy on the part of the girls who aren't developing quite as fast as you.

So don't worry. You'll find that breasts are nice to have, in more ways than one.

First, they have a definite use. If one day you have a baby, your breasts will produce and store the milk that is your baby's first food. (Nowadays, many babies are fed from a bottle instead, but nature provides mother's milk as well.)

Long before you start having babies, though, you'll find that breasts help you look pretty good. Boys and men like them a lot, and quite right too. Breasts are part of what makes you look different from men and attractive to them.

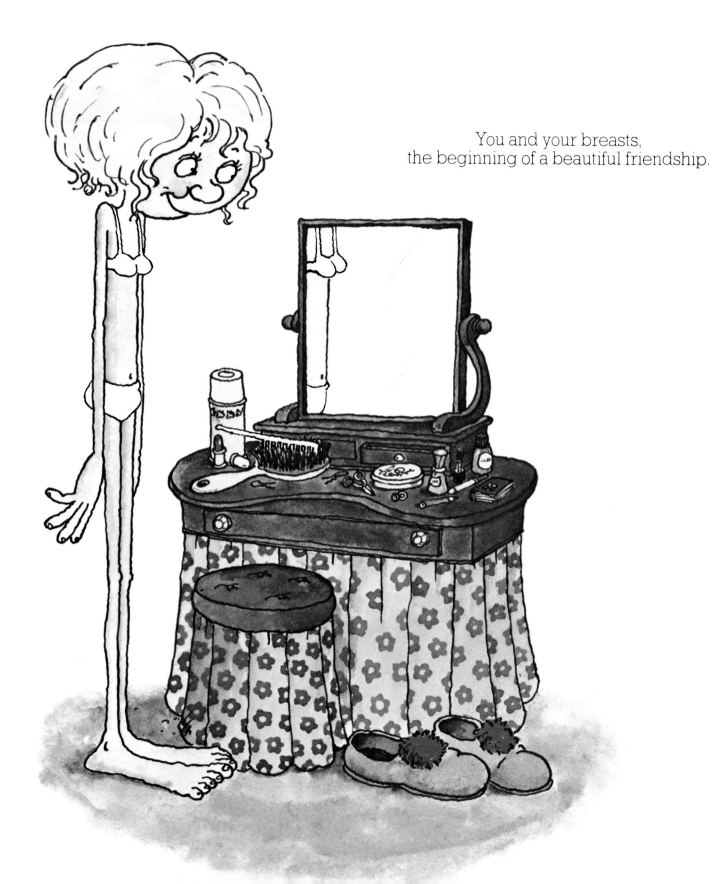

You and your breasts,
the beginning of a beautiful friendship.

Here's something else you'll notice about breasts. Next time you go out, take a look at the women you see walking along the street.

Their breasts come in many shapes and sizes: big ones, small ones, high ones, low ones, melon-shaped, pear-shaped, pointed, flat, and so on.

But every breast, however different in shape, has a nipple.

This is the small, slightly darker part on the tip of each breast, and it's usually the most sensitive part of the breast. Being so sensitive, touching it or having it touched gently can give you a very nice feeling.

Nice as that can be, however, it's not the only reason you have nipples. Nature put them there to act as milk faucets for your baby. The nipple is the place where mother's milk actually comes out of the breast.

When does breast development begin? Well, it can start any time between the ages of eight and thirteen. When isn't important. The important thing is that you're happy to have them.

All sizes and all shapes are attractive to the opposite sex. Big ones are beautiful; small ones are beautiful. Breasts are lovely and useful parts of your body. Be proud of them.

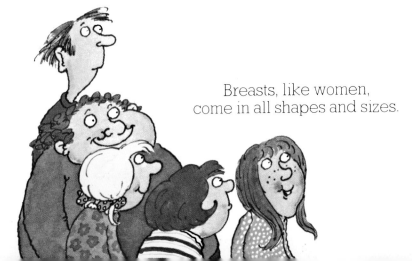

Breasts, like women, come in all shapes and sizes.

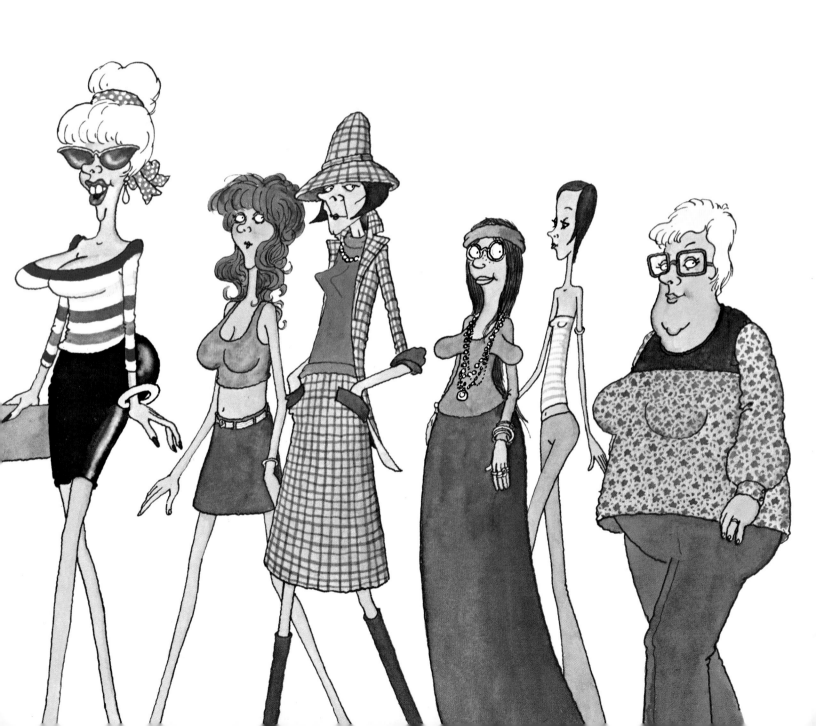

## "What's an erection?"

If you're a boy, you have something in common with every other boy. You have a penis.

When your penis gets stiff, it becomes bigger than usual. That's called an erection.

You won't remember your first erection. It probably happened when you were just a few weeks or months old. Since then, your penis has taken it easy, and you've only had erections at odd intervals. But now you'll notice that it begins to happen more and more often.

Sometimes you get an erection for no reason at all. Other times it happens because you see a girl and start thinking about how it would feel to touch her or kiss her.

Most erections, then, begin in your head because of something you're thinking. This causes extra blood to rush from other parts of your body into your penis. And that's why it becomes bigger and stiffer than usual.

You may wonder why the extra blood comes to your penis rather than, for instance, your big toe.

Well, the area round your penis has suddenly become very, very active. Amazing and wonderful things are happening.

Under your penis is a small bag of skin containing your testicles (usually called balls). There are two of them, and they're busy. They're producing sperm and they're producing testosterone.

Testosterone as you've read, is the male sex hormone. It makes your pubic hair grow and your voice get deeper.

Semen is the fluid that carries sperm. And sperm make babies when they join up with the woman's eggs.

For most of the time, though, your sperm are inside your body, waiting and twiddling their thumbs. What they'd really like to do is get out.

Sperm can't do very much except sit around until you get an erection.

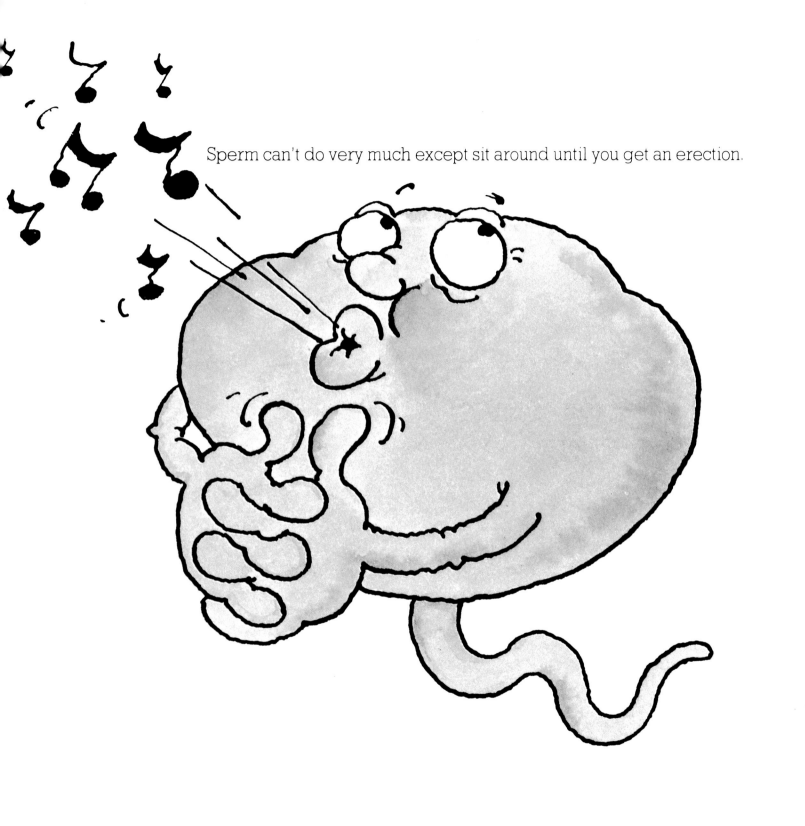

Now, there's only one exit for the sperm; through the hole at the end of your penis. (When your penis is soft, that's the hole you urinate through. But when it's erect, it's the way out for the sperm-carrying semen that travels up in special tubes from testicles.) So really, an erection is your sperm telling you they want to come out.

That's all. It's normal, it's natural and very soon you'll find that releasing the semen (which is called ejaculating or "coming") is a very pleasurable feeling.

One last word about erections. They sometimes happen just at the moment when you wish they wouldn't. Like at the swimming pool, or when you have to stand up in class.

Don't panic. Try to think about something else. When your penis realizes you're not interested in it the erection will go.

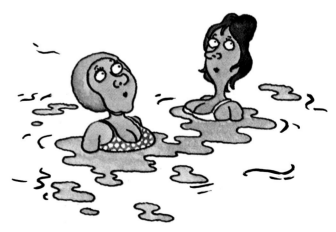

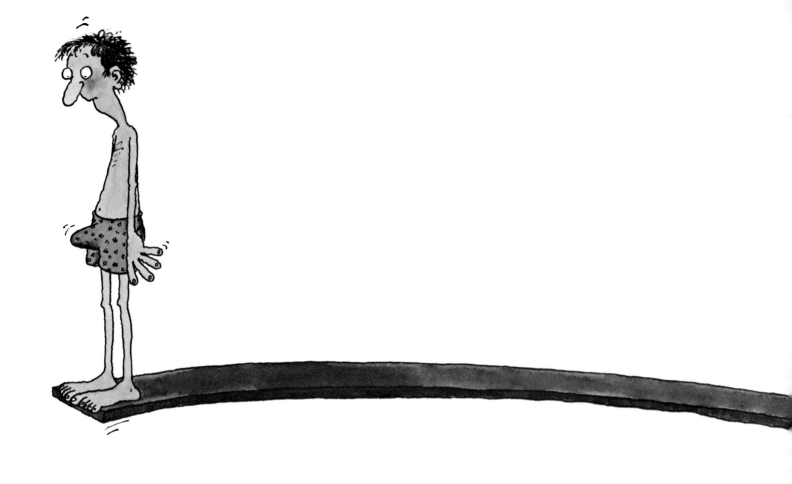

Erections sometimes don't know when they're not wanted.

## "What's a period?"

A girl's first period can come as quite a shock.

It normally happens around twelve or thirteen, and it can come without any warning. You could be sitting in the movies, or at school, or you could wake up one morning and find some blood between your legs. Just like that.

As you can imagine, this could be frightening if you didn't anticipate it and know what it was.

The blood, of course, comes from inside you and out through your vagina. But before explaining why, there are a few general facts about periods you should know.

At the time of your period, you may have a stomachache or you may feel nothing. Sometimes for months before their first period, girls have vague abdominal pains, or feel sleepy, or irritable. That usually clears up, as if by magic, after you've had two or three normal periods.

Dr. Earl M. Cooperman of Ottawa, Canada, reminds us to say that periods are often irregular in time and duration for the first year they occur.

He adds: "It is best for girls to dismiss the warnings of their well meaning relatives about 'the curse' and accept the discomforts of menses (the period) as a small inconvenient fact of life."

Another fact of life is that periods are a very necessary part of being a woman. To understand why, you need to know about your womb.

Your womb is where a baby lives for the nine months it develops inside your body. Most of the time, obviously, you haven't got a baby inside you. But your body gets prepared, just in case.

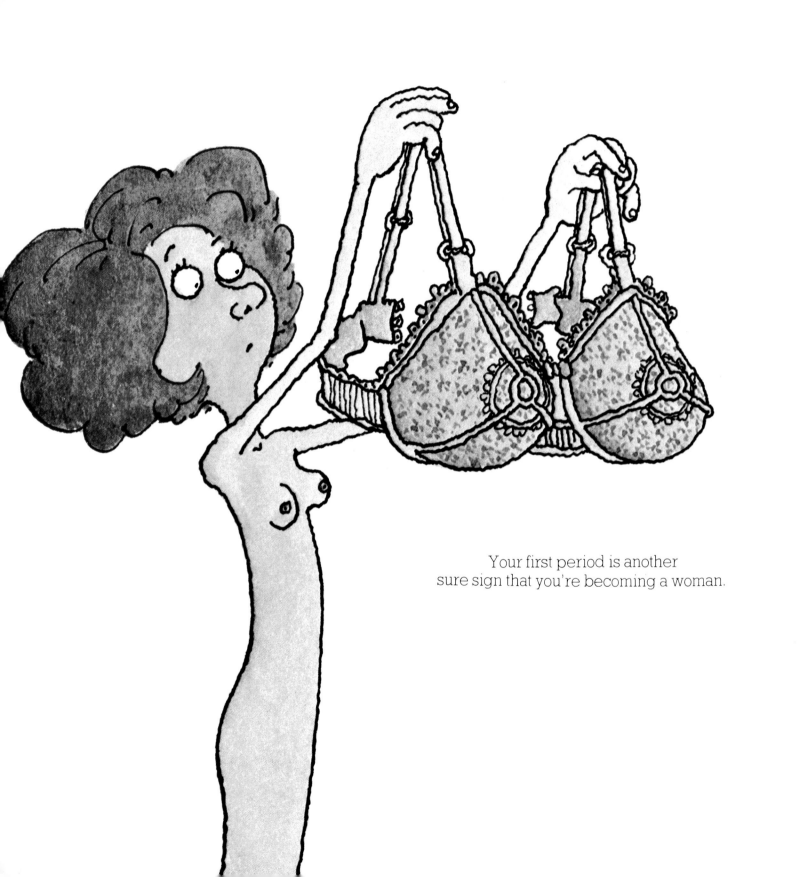

Your first period is another
sure sign that you're becoming a woman.

Every month, you make inside yourself a new lining for your womb, to be ready for a baby if you should start to make one. You also produce eggs which are microscopic in size. These wait for their male counterparts, the sperm, to fertilize them.

And every month, the old lining and the unfertilized eggs have to come out to make room for the new ones.

This all comes out, as you know by now, between your legs in the form of blood.

How come you don't notice when other women are having their periods? They either wear a pad or something called a tampon that absorbs the blood. (A tampon is worn inside the vagina. It's neat, and most girls hardly feel it.) Once you start having regular periods, that's what you'll use too. It's convenient, it's effective, and it lets you do pretty much everything you would normally do-even go swimming.

The process of having a period happens on an average of once every 28 days, although that can vary from person to person. The proper name for this is the Menstrual Cycle, and discharging blood is called menstruating.

Whatever you call it and however long it takes to happen, you'll be startled by it at first. But you'll get used to those few inconvenient days each month, even though they may sometimes make you a little depressed and grouchy.

There's no getting away from the fact that periods are more of a chore than a pleasure. But they're a very necessary part of growing up to be a woman. After all, if you didn't have periods, you couldn't have children.

Don't worry if your periods don't come smack on the 28th day. The timing cycle varies from woman to woman.

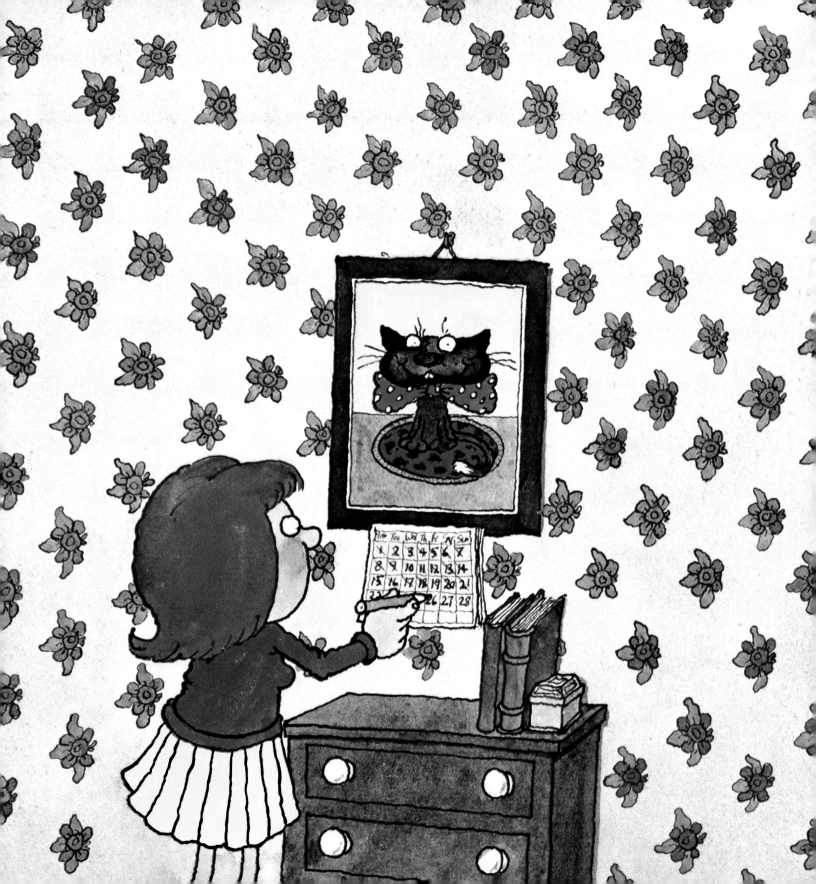

## "Why is my voice acting so funny?"

There comes a time in every young man's life when his voice starts playing tricks on him.

The tricks are caused by the larynx and vocal cords getting bigger. This affects the voice, making it "break."

It should happen to you when you're about thirteen or fourteen, and for some months you may actually have two voices. Your child's voice, which is high. And your man's voice, which is much deeper.

The trouble is, there's a short time when you're never quite sure which one is going to come out when you open your mouth. You can even go from high to low (or vice versa) in one sentence.

While this is happening, you may feel that everybody must be listening to hear your voice go from squeaky to deep.

They're not. And once your new voice settles in, you can relax. It won't change again, and your squeaking days will be over.

The day your voice breaks, you won't be able to reach those high notes any more.

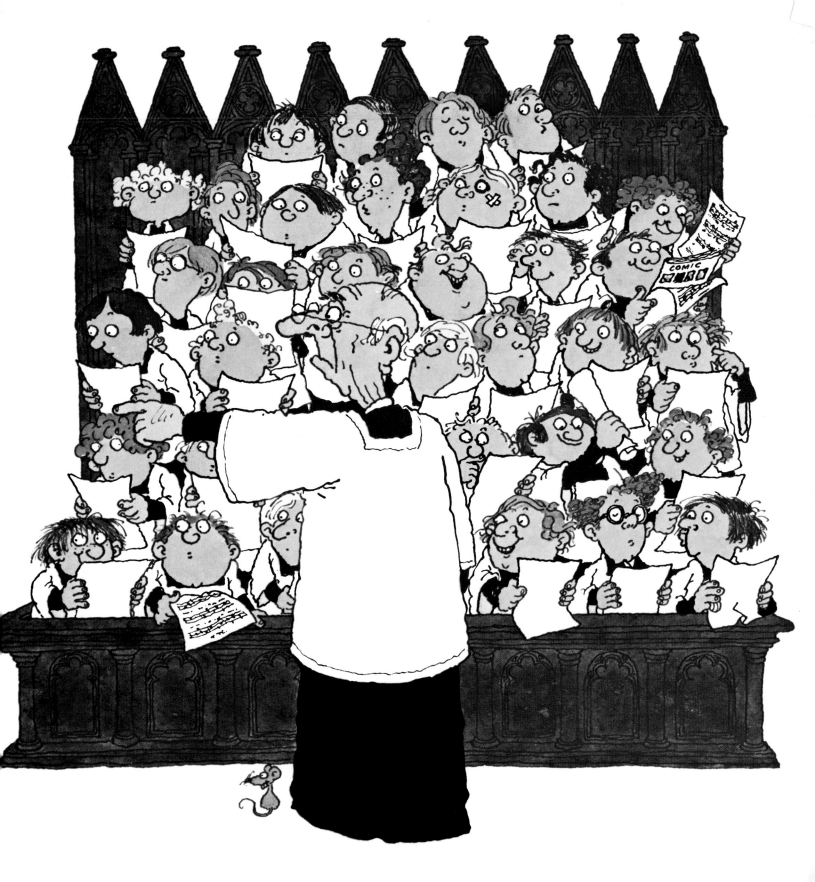

## "Why do I get pimples?"

Both girls and boys get them. And whether you call them pimples or spots or acne, they're something you can certainly do without.

A few lucky people grow up without ever having a pimple rear its ugly head. But they're rare. Most of us have to put up with them for a year or two.

It's a dirty trick on nature's part, because it usually happens just about the time when you're getting interested in the opposite sex. There you are, hoping to look as attractive as you can, when along comes a pimple.

Yet, strangely enough, pimples are caused by something that's good for the skin.

By the time you're thirteen or fourteen, your hormones are working overtime on your sebaceous glands. (That's pronounced seb-ayshus.)

These glands live in your skin. Their job is to produce a kind of thick oil that keeps your skin supple and healthy, and prevents it from drying up.

Unfortunately, during this particular time of your life, your sebaceous glands get very enthusiastic and produce far more oil than your skin needs.

This extra oil gets stuck in the tiny holes in your skin called pores; then a speck of dirt gets stuck there, too. Next thing you know, you're the not too proud owner of a pimple.

Pimples often happen when you become a big oil producer

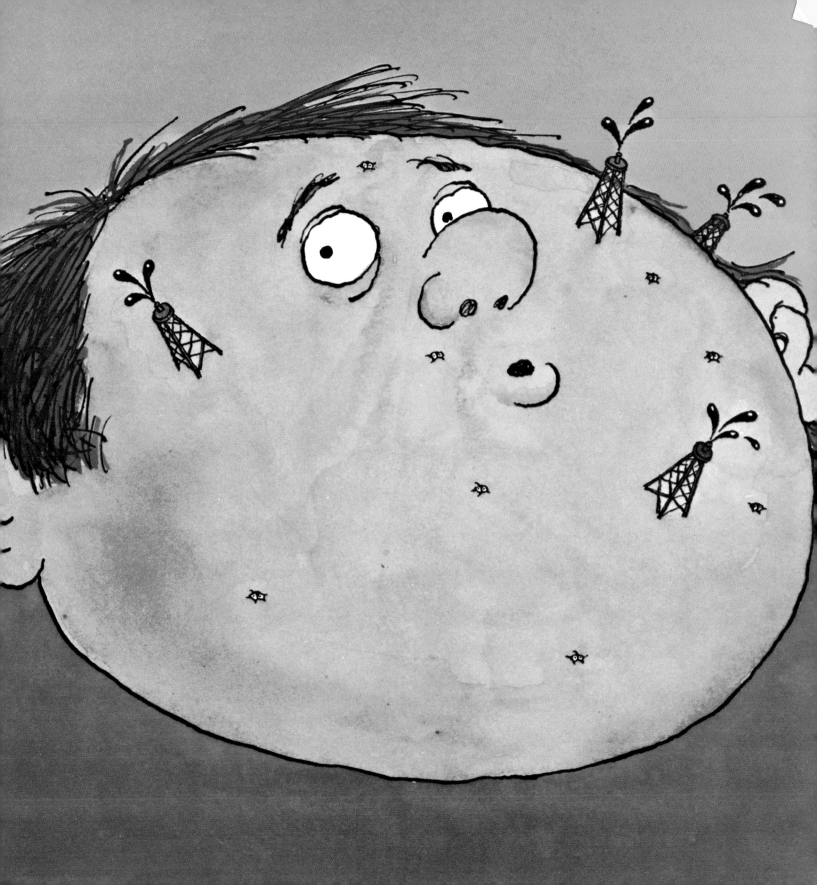

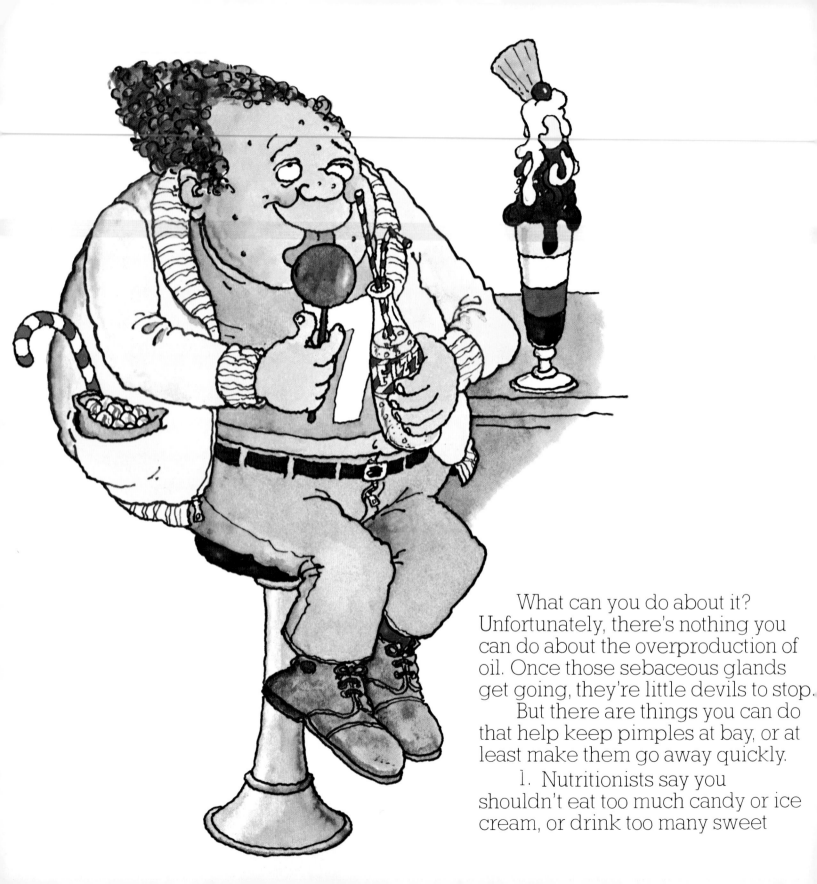

What can you do about it? Unfortunately, there's nothing you can do about the overproduction of oil. Once those sebaceous glands get going, they're little devils to stop.

But there are things you can do that help keep pimples at bay, or at least make them go away quickly.

1. Nutritionists say you shouldn't eat too much candy or ice cream, or drink too many sweet

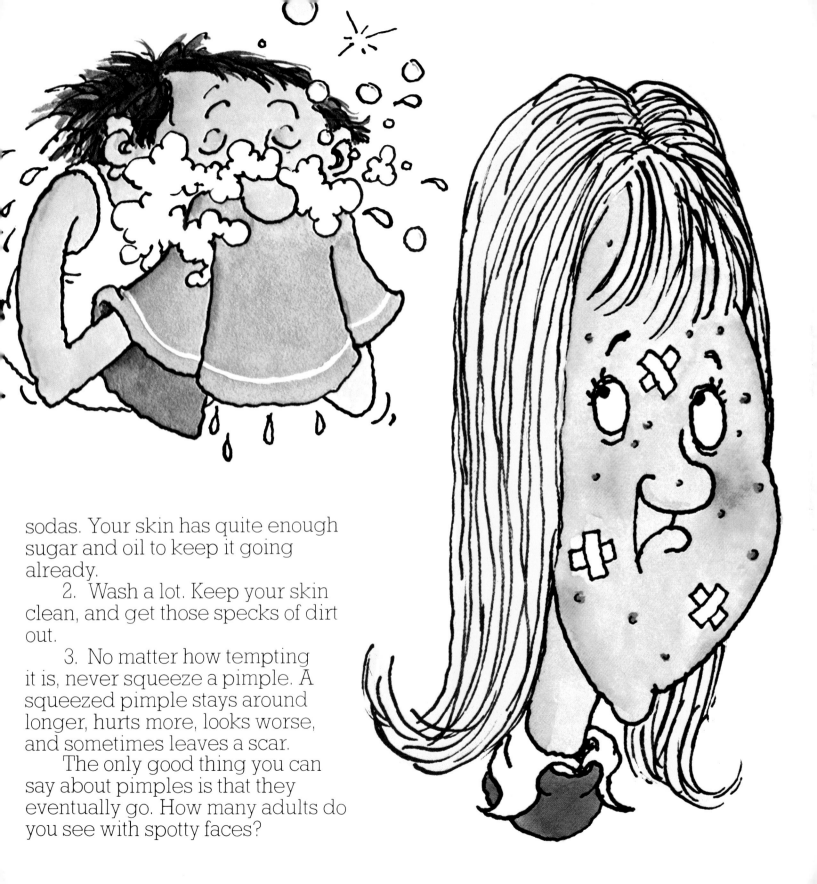

sodas. Your skin has quite enough sugar and oil to keep it going already.

2. Wash a lot. Keep your skin clean, and get those specks of dirt out.

3. No matter how tempting it is, never squeeze a pimple. A squeezed pimple stays around longer, hurts more, looks worse, and sometimes leaves a scar.

The only good thing you can say about pimples is that they eventually go. How many adults do you see with spotty faces?

### "What's masturbation?"

If, when you were younger, you read "Where Did I Come From?," or some other good book on the subject, you know some of the facts of life. If you don't know them, it's time to learn.

Our civilization is an advanced one. And in advanced cultures, mating is done later in life so that the young have more time to educate themselves.

That's fine. Except that by the age of thirteen or so, your body is ready for mating. Physically, you can have children. Mentally and socially, you're not ready to have them yet.

So nature has created her own solution. It's called masturbation. Men do it. Women do it. Even some animals do it. It's a way of getting sexual release without the full act of mating with a member of the opposite sex.

(Mating at too early an age is a mistake. You should first learn about birth control methods and how to use them. Also, about venereal disease and how to avoid it. Your doctor can give you good advice about both.)

You'll hear all kinds of strange stories about masturbation: that it makes you go blind, it makes you go crazy, or even that it makes hair grow on the palms of your hands.

It does none of these things.

It's a perfectly healthy and normal function.

Masturbation is usually your first sexual experience. It's sometimes called "playing with yourself." Girls use their fingers to caress and rub their vagina and clitoris (a small but very sensitive area just above the entrance of your vagina). Boys do the same with their penis.

This usually starts because you're thinking more and more about the opposite sex. Your imagination creates scenes that

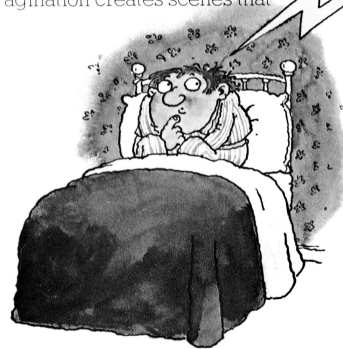

cause you to become sexually excited, sexual tension builds up, and that's when you get the urge to touch and play with yourself.

If you rub and caress long enough, you'll have an orgasm. This is a release of the sexual excitement that has built up inside you. And it's a great feeling.

To repeat: masturbation is a normal, healthy part of growing up.

Don't worry. Nothing dreadful happens when you masturbate.

Don't let anyone try to make you feel guilty about it. (If they do, suggest that they read Sex Without Guilt by Dr. Albert Ellis; especially his first chapter, "New Light on Masturbation.")

We're not suggesting that you take up nonstop masturbating. For one thing, your body won't cooperate. And, like everything else, if you do it to excess, it becomes boring.

But masturbation doesn't have any bad effects, and it doesn't hurt anybody. So let it make you feel good, not guilty.

## "Why am I getting hairy?"

With girls, it starts growing around eleven or twelve. With boys, about thirteen or fourteen.

"It" is hair. The kind that grows on your face (if you're a boy), under your arms, and between your legs. This last kind is called pubic hair, because it grows on the pubes.

The only problem about pubic hair is that both girls and boys sometimes get hung up about it. They think they either have too much or too little.

In fact, there's no such thing as the perfect amount of pubic hair. We all have our own little patch. Whether yours is larger or thicker or darker than your friend's doesn't matter at all.

Whatever color or thickness it is, pubic hair can often be attractive to the opposite sex. It acts as a kind of magnetic field for sexual stimulation. That, and to provide your genitals with a certain amount of protection, is why it's there.

One last thing. Don't worry if your pubic hair doesn't match the color of the hair on your head. It often happens that they're not the same shade. If that's the case with you, don't think you're odd.

You're absolutely normal, but maybe a shade more interesting.

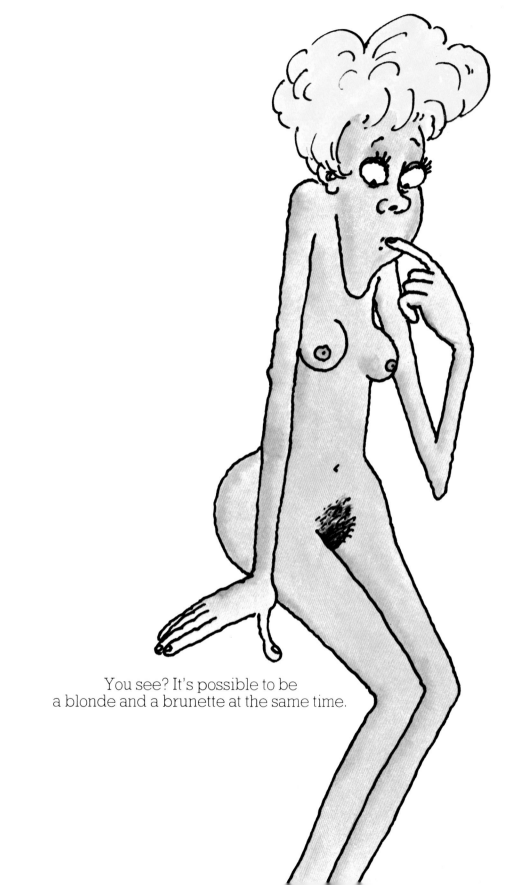

You see? It's possible to be
a blonde and a brunette at the same time.

### "What's a wet dream?"

You remember that we described earlier how sperm get out of a boy's body? Well, masturbation is one way out; wet dreams are another.

Wet dreams start when you're maybe thirteen or fourteen. As you'd expect from the name, they happen when you're asleep.

The sperm that you have been making reach a level where they just have to get out. And if you don't let them out by masturbating, they wait till you're asleep and shoot out by themselves.

It sounds simple, but there's more to it than that. For a start, very little sperm can escape unless you have an erection. And, remember, when all this happens you're sleeping.

So first, you have a night-time erection which is often caused by a specially pleasant dream.

Perhaps your dream is about a girl you know, or a photograph you saw in a magazine. Or maybe it's about a nice feeling you had when you were awake.

The result is that you get an erection, have an orgasm, the sperm shoot out, and you wake up with sticky pajamas.

There's only one thing wrong with wet dreams; you're not awake to enjoy them.

(Girls, incidentally, have fewer wet dreams and many have none at all. But to make up for that, a girl can often masturbate many more times a day than a boy.)

Wet dreams feel much better th. ordinary dreams. No wonder he's smilir

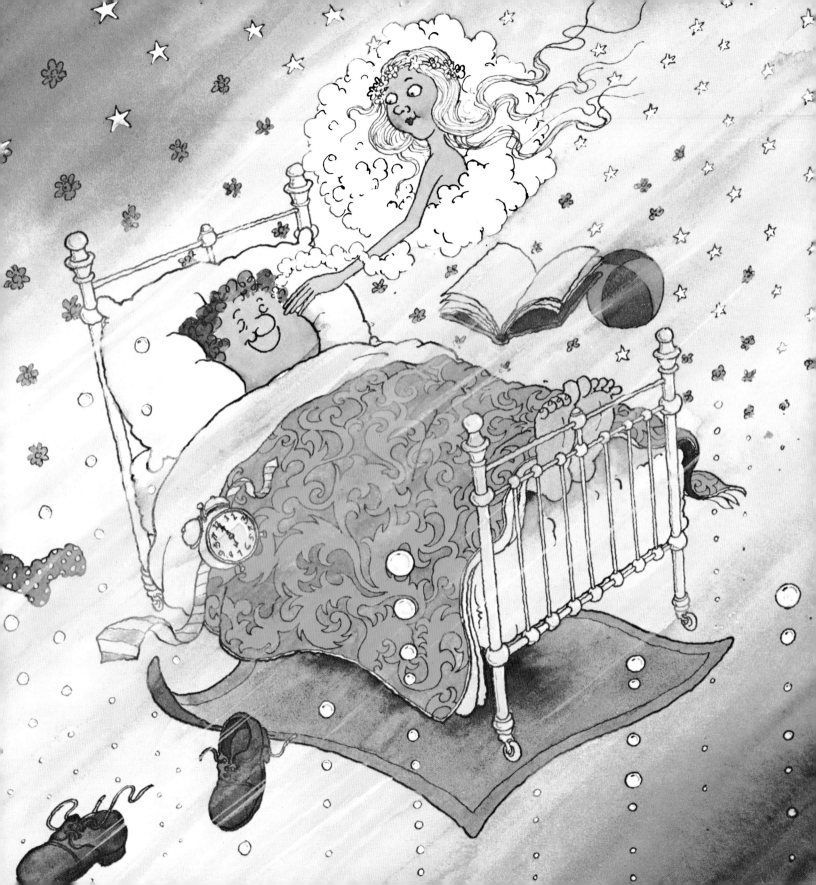

## "Why is mine not like his?"

A lot of you boys may have done this already. But if you haven't, do it. Take a look at some other boys' penises.

You'll see that there are two different kinds.

One is the kind where the outer layer of skin (called the foreskin) covers the whole of the penis.

The other kind is where the foreskin stops just before the end of the penis. There's a special name for how the second kind got that way: circumcision.

This is a bit of minor surgery done while you're still an infant. The doctor who does it just snips off that skin hat, leaving the end of the penis bare.

Circumcision started hundreds and hundreds of years ago. It's still an important ritual in the Jewish religion as well as in many others.

More recently, some doctors have circumcised boys for health reasons rather than religious ones. Other doctors disagree. There is no rule and no proof that either way is better than the other.

If you happen to be circumcised, fine. It's every bit as good as the other way, and it may be slightly easier for you to keep your penis clean. But circumcision doesn't affect the size of the penis or anything else.

And while we're on the subject of size, here's an interesting fact about penises.

Despite what other boys may tell you, the majority of penises are about the same size when they're erect. In a fully grown man, that's between six and seven inches. (Although, obviously, there are longer and shorter exceptions.)

Another myth is that a bigger penis is a better penis. Experienced women will tell you that this just isn't so. It's not how big it is, but what you do with it that counts when you're making love.

Many "great lovers" had small penises. And many men with over-size penises are washouts as lovers.

The time when you notice the difference in size of penises most is when they aren't erect. You'll see next time you're in a shower room with a lot of other boys.

But the differences can be very misleading. Because the bigger the penis is when it isn't erect, the less it usually grows when it is erect, and vice versa. The important thing is how big your penis is

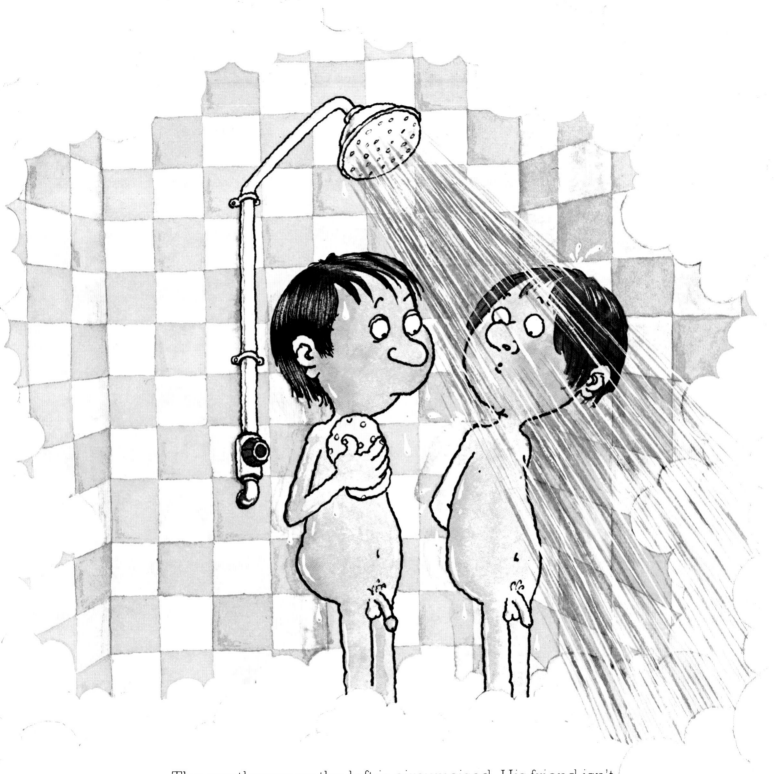

The gentleman on the left is circumcised. His friend isn't.

when it's erect. And, as we've said, when penises are erect, they're more or less equal in length.

It's interesting to know that girls are built differently, too. The vagina can be positioned higher or lower. The pubic hair can be diamond shaped or heart shaped. The clitoris stands out, or can be enfolded by soft skin.

But, like penises, one healthy vagina has all the attributes of any other healthy vagina. They may look different, but they can all give and receive the same pleasure.

## "What happens next?"

We hope we've answered some of the big questions. If we have left some things unanswered, don't be afraid to ask someone you trust. And never forget that what you're going through is part of the experience of living and growth.

Once you come through puberty, rather like a consolation prize, you get into what should be one of the happiest times of your life.

The greatest thing that can happen to you will probably happen during those next few years.

You'll meet someone and you'll fall in love.

Part of falling in love is sex. When love and sex are combined, they make up what has to be one of the best feelings in the world.

Enjoy it. Take good care of yourself. And good luck.

And so we say goodbye to pubert

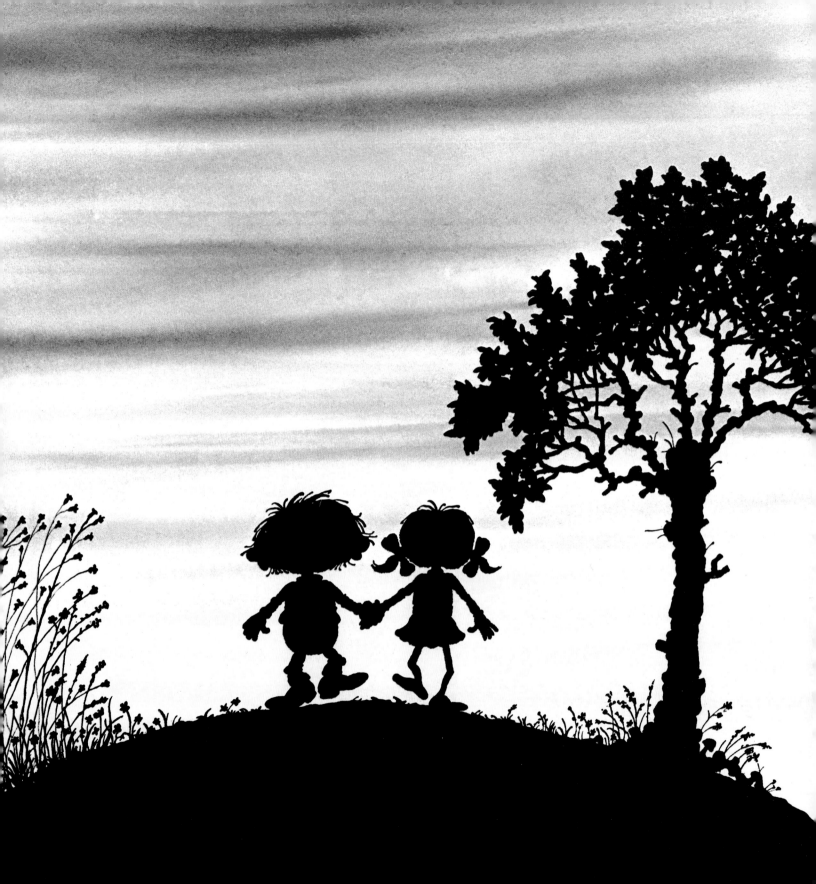